I0705090

100% You

By Sammy Moorman

Table of Contents

Contact the author
sammybooks911@gmail.com

Thank you to everyone that was a part of my journey.
S.M.

Be a better you
Feel better
Look better
Let the real you out
That voice hidden inside of that beautiful mind. let it out!

Take control. Use the secret power of 100. The power of you. You will slowly build a strong mind, body and soul. A simple solution for a Big problem.

Chapter 1
Let's Go!

We are all going through something. Our minds are too distracted. Refocus on what really matters. You. I'll be with you for your whole journey. I started my journey sad, confused with slight focused. Excuse after excuses, that's all I was hearing. Shut up! Stop blaming everything or everyone. Accept truth. The problem is you. Look in the mirror. Tell yourself who you want to be. Say it. Say it often. Say it loud. Get your main goal in your positive mind. The world will start to give you signs your doing the right thing. Going for a dream.

A Dream can be anything. Financial body, job, love or a new car. Any dream you have you can create. First step of using the power of 100% You. Is you!! You need yourself remember that all you got. Yes some of us do have a great support network. The main captain of this ship is you. No matter what waters the ship is going through the captain stays at the wheel. Control yourself. Stay strong mentally. Stay focused. You have a goal and a dream. Go do it! No one else will. You have made up your mind. You've seen your dream you have your goal. Now it's time to make it happen. The power of 100% You begins.

Chapter 2
Attitude

Attitude is everything. A positive attitude can change the whole world. It's easy to get down on yourself. Trust me, I know I've pulled up from it found, the best version of myself. Search and find the things that help you succeed to be better. Anything you are excellent at. Embrace it. Go for it do it. Accomplish something. It doesn't matter, you know what you're a true master of. Let it out. We've been hiding our true abilities, powers and gifts for a long me. It's time let you be you. Allow yourself to grow show your gift to everyone. Don't forget not everyone has your magical gift. Some people are great talker. Some people are great performers. Others are great pizza makers some are great athletes, amazing business people great CPAs. Whatever you're good at just have fun with it. Bring a positive attitude to every situation. Even if it's not positive just smile a little bit. That smile can help. Don't be shy say hello to people. A rule I use and live by is the 5-10 feet rule. If someone's 5 feet to 10 feet from you just say hello, Say how you doing? Go have some fun today. Spread positivity. The positivity will spread back to you. Be positive in your journey, you're about to finish strong.

Taking that positive attitude in to a work out mind set. In any working out activity always take the mindset of 100. 100 reps and once you've surpassed the hundred go into 200, 300, 400 and more. Keep on growing you becoming a master at your craft, and that craft is you. You deserve more than anyone else in this world, so give yourself what you deserve. Go for it!Make it happen, be a dreamer be a believer, be you use that power. Represent yourself the way you need to be represented. We've all been hiding for way too long. It's time to show yourself to yourself. Enjoy. Be happy. Be 100 times better. Be 100% YOU!!

Chapter 3
Goals

You can do it. Give yourself a goal. Start Small even if it's losing 5 pounds. That's fine whatever you want. It's your personal goal, now go for it and do it. The biggest gift to yourself is getting your goals accomplished. Granted once you succeed. You will feel a sense of relief a sense of achievement, a sense of awesomeness, a sense of knowing how great you truly are! Wow! I can do this. Yes you can. Yes I Can. You're the only one that can be the better version of yourself. You're in there let it out. I want you to write your goals down. Say them out loud every morning in the mirror, in the shower or on the commode. The car ride into work. Even in negative situations or work out struggles. Just say. I'm doing this for this you get that goal in. Alex Morgan mind set. SCORE! You will win! You will achieve! You can do anything you just have to try. If you don't get it the first time try again. I bet after a 100 times you get it! Don't stop believing in yourself. Believe your dreams. They were given to you. You only. You can achieve them. Go for them don't forget them. Now say it out loud. Whatever that dream and goal is. Say it proudly scream it. Believe it, Go make it happen!

Chapter 4
Motivation

Find your motivation. Now that can be hard. There's a lot of days I personally feel like I don't wanna do nothing, that's when you gotta smack yourself in the face. Look in the mirror and say let's go baby! You can do this. Find a source of motivation. This could sound silly to some. It doesn't matter whatever motivates you motivates you. You could watch the ultimate warrior running in the ring and wrestling the honky-tonk man. Your favorite scene in Gladiator. Singing your favorite Taylor Swift song. You could look at your child, that can motivate you. Whatever you need to hear you do it. Listen dream and achieve. find what helps you motivated. If watching sports and listening to Curren$y helps you motivate. Then do it! Simple. Whatever you need to help you get your goals and motivate you. Something else you could do take a picture of whatever your dream is. Put it right above your bed. When you wake up you see it. When you go to sleep you see it. Your dream and motivation is right there and do it. Just find the motivation Listen to Arnold Schwarzenegger give his rules of success listen to. Les Brown find a motivational key and use that key. It unlocks more than you can imagine. The motivation helps you when you need your extra push. You're doing it. Sometimes we need just a little bit of help.

Chapter 5
Change

Change is ultimately going to happen. You are personally going to change. Your clothes are gonna change. Your attitude is going to change, you're becoming better in every way. Change is OK. Change for the better never change for the worse. If you find yourself in a situation of change of the worse. Change it! Only you can change it. Find the positive. Positive way to get out of your negative situation and change it for the better. You are the best solution for positive change, your whole world is going to change as you become the person that you were meant to be. That you've always have been. Let the change happen, Embrace it, maybe you can change the world.

Chapter 6
Honesty

Be honest to yourself. Be a realist. You have to be honest with yourself. You have to look at all your situations. Look yourself in the mirror. You have to know you're good and you're bad. Oh chores your best attributes as well. You have to be honest with yourself. If you're in a really bad situation and your life really can't get better because of that situation. Be honest with yourself and get out! Now stop wasting time. We don't get much time in this crazy place. Get out of Bad relationships Bad jobs Bad whatever. If it's not working. Get out of it, you're better than this. Yes you are. You don't need this. If you're living a different life to become a better person and if anyone around you is not always becoming better. Then why are you there? Be honest with yourself. Look at your friends look at your family. If you're not getting support you need. Its ok to grow alone. You may be alone during this journey. That's OK. That's why we're all here together. We are here to accomplish something. We all need to improve in our daily lives. That's why we're doing this. It might be to lose 5,10 pounds or 300 pounds or just to try something different. Boredom. Just be honest with yourself. When you look in the mirror you know what's true and what's not. What you believe in stick with it. Get your goal, make it happen. You're the only one that can be honest with yourself, You will thank yourself later.

Chapter 7
Praise and cleanse

Praise yourself!
Congratulate yourself on little victories. Congratulate yourself all the time. Let
yourself know that you love yourself. You have to be the best version you can be.
That starts simple, when you're taking a shower in the morning. Smile while you're in
the shower, it helps listen to something positive that keeps you going first thing in the
morning. By letting the positivity in and praising yourself you start to give yourself
confidence. Cleansing yourself. Praising yourself you bring a good aura into areas.
People know that you are just all around good person. Positive attitude, smelling good
being sharp, working hard. That's a lot better than the other, Take pride in yourself
cleanse yourself, brush your teeth wash your hair, wash your body find an every day
scent get a perfume or cologne. Explore find a personal scent that fits you. One that
expresses your personality that you love. It will become a part of you. Just don't
forget to congratulate yourself. You're doing AWESOME! Keep on doing great
things.

Chapter 8
-Wins

Everyone needs a win. It's easy to win. Small victories lead to big wins. Start Small. Simply if you can get one more set while working out that's a win. If you can fast for 15 more minutes, that's a win. If you can drink more water than you have in one day than you did all month that's a win. You walked all the way to the end of your street that's a win! Your little wins will equal a huge victory at the end. Don't stop keep fighting congratulate yourself. It's terrible when you're down and out. When you haven't gotten a win in a while, small wins will help build you up. So you better be ready for the victory! Take every small positive affirmation and turn it into more positivity in your life. You will win! Just say it. I will win. Some wins takes time. Don't be scared. Don't be shy. Go get it. Make it happen. You're a winner and always will be! "Just Win, baby". Al Davis Raiders owner

Chapter 9
Workout

Great job! You took the first step. Now let's talk about the workout plan to tackle
your goal. Got the workout clothes on. Now looking around the gym or your home
saying. What am I doing? You're kicking ASS! That's what you're doing. Like I said
I'm here with you through your journey. Now your thinking where do I start. Easy…
Yes it's all about the power of 100. 100% every time. You can do it. Start slow.
Former athletes former fast food drive thru order champions let's begin.
Consult with your doctor before beginning a diet and workout regiment.
First Work outs
Beginners start with 10 reps one set.
Proceed on each exercise until you feel confident and comfortable to push yourself to
the next set goals. Until you reach the hundred.
Start with 10 reps 10 times (sets)
Squats
no weight just your body weight. Standing in front of a chair or bench. Slowly move
your knees until your rear end touches the chair or bench. After touching the bench or
chair. Fire up fast or your own pace to a standing straight up to slowly back down to
the chair or bench. You will feel the work in your hamstrings thighs, lower back
buttocks and calves.
10 reps 10 times =100
If you feel comfortable go for it! do 25 reps 4 times.
Remember by doing and using the power of 100%. You will do more than you have
ever done. It sounds intimidating 100 reps. It is. Once you have successfully
completed it. You already did more than last year.
-push ups
Any way you feel comfortable kneeling on the ground to different elevations. Find
your comfort zone. Even if you never done a push up. Just try. You can do anything.

-Beginning start with the 10x10
Any push-up position. If you feel your position is too easy them switch to a more
intermediate position push-up option.
-25x4 10x10 50x2 whatever you feel comfortable at do it. Just get the 100 reps in.

-sit ups /crunches/ leg lifts/ bicycle kicks
Same formula as our other exercises.
10x10 25x4 50x2
bicycle kicks- ride that bike in the air. Any speed you can. Keep your feet in the air.
Do not touch the ground. Feeling the burn in your core and legs

Lying on your back. Legs up in a position that resembles riding a bike. Kick and move them legs in a peddling motion. Never touching the ground.
Leg lifts.
Laying flat on your back hold your legs up in the air 1-2 feet from the ground. Holding the position. Feeling your core working. Hold the position for 10-100 seconds.
-Hip Thrust
Laying flat with your knees up at a 90degree angle. Slowly move your hip/pelvis up to the sky. Feeling the muscles work in your hamstring, buttocks glutes and abs. Grow that booty. Same repetition.
-10x10 25x4 50x2 for more advanced users you can add weights such as a barbells. Increase speed or decrease speed whatever feels best and grows your muscles pushing yourself to new limits.

Consult with your doctor before doing a diet and workout regiment.

Chapter 10
-Cardio

Just like the rest of our exercise. Start doing 10 minutes walking/running/elliptical whatever works best for your body. Walk around your neighborhood. Go explore the world around you. Now every day try to add one more minute. Each time you do your cardio. You will slowly get better and feel better that's the most important part. You can do your cardio anyway you want on the same days as your exercise or your off day. Start with 10 minutes and see where you finish. It becomes a game with yourself. Set that timer. Get to MOVING!! Explore the world around you. It's waiting.

Yes, it seems like a lot at first.
Now take your time. If you can only do 10 crunches, leg lifts, push-ups whatever. That's fine. If it takes you all day to do 100. you do 10 when you can. Wake up do 10. take a break at work do 10. Takes three hours to run errands do 10. Do whatever you gotta do. 10 reps or more anytime you can. as long as you hit the hundred plateau in a day you have succeeded, you have won.
Start small if you can't do the 100 starting off. Just start with 10-25 then go to 50 then 75. Then boom you reached it. Take your time but PUSH YOURSELF!!

Now, this particular one can get a little crazy. First your gonna to push yourself on this one harder than you've pushed yourself on anything else before. This will not take as long as the others. Your going to do this fast as possible. You can push yourself remember when you're done, you're gonna do more in this one session then you've done all year. You're gonna do more in this one session than your neighbor has done in two years. The power of 100! You can do it. You're the best now go for it. You will do your sit ups or crunches whatever feels best for you. I prefer crunches after doing your first set you will not take a break you will immediately go into leg-lifts or bicycle kicks for 10 seconds 25 seconds 50 seconds or 100 seconds whatever feels best for your body, once you've done the 10 to 25 seconds of the leg lifts or bicycle kicks, go back into the crunch as fast as you can do this again. After the third set you may take a break for one minute once that one minute has hit go strong and finish your last two sets! If you're doing the 10 x 10 method after every two sets and two leg lifts or bicycle kicks you may take your one minute break. The goal is to do the sit-ups and leg lifts for a full core workout as much as you can do in a little amount of time. It's to shock your body to make you better, your core is your whole body. This may be the hardest exercise for any of us to overcome this is the one that's going to push you this is gonna have the one that you're gonna feel it from your stomach, your hips your legs to your toes. You will feel your leg lifts and bicycle kicks like no other, you're gonna feel pain and tension just remember it's weakness leaving your body. Your stronger than you even know. You're the best and you can do it. Remember after your hundred sets or your seconds of leg-lifts and whatnot you've already done more than you've done in a year! Great Job Rockstar!

These four exercising and walks two - three times a week will help you benefit mentally, physically better then you've ever felt before. You are the captain of the ship so let's take this ship to our destination! Where you want to go? You can do anything you can be everything. Just have to go for it and do it. Yes there's gonna be tough times there's gonna be rough days but guess what? Wipe them rough moments away, you keep on going Cause I guarantee you after 100 days of doing this power of 100 you will feel 100 times better than you have ever felt. live by the power of 100 do it all! Once you've gotten past the power of 100 you go into 200, 300, 400, 100000 it just keeps on going and you keep on growing to become a better human, Than you ever thought you could be. Do it do it! You're the problem. You're the answer. You're the solution. Now go do it!! The world's waiting.

This is just the beginning of the exercise. Of course. You can do different exercise, routines, and machines whatever you wanna do to strengthen the areas of your body and muscles. There is no wrong or right way. The main goal. The main focus of this lifestyle is doing 100 reps of one particular exercise so once you've done multiple exercises you have done over 500 to 1000 reps. Totally shocking your body and making you become stronger leaner and just feeling better. That's all that really matters.

Chapter 11
Diets

This is where people can call my idea crazy. I don't believe in doing an extreme diet. I believe in you. Doing what makes you happy because that's what the power of 100 is. About you feeling your best and being happy. Take a multivitamin. Do what works for you. Make better choices on what you eat if you. Personally when I starting this journey, did it by fasting I would drink water and 1 energy drink. You can have any energy drink, pre-workout black coffee. Any beverage that helps motivate you in the morning that has less than 25 calories. Lots and Lots of water throughout the day, but the big helpful change was I would not ingest any food until 3 PM or 5 PM. If I could go later, I would go later. I learned by doing this I felt better. My body started to heal itself I had knee problems, shoulder pains stomach issues. They slowly all went away. The fasting, the working out shocking the body this way, putting a new lifestyle in is easy and hard for you. The easy part about it is. You really don't have to change your diet at all. Still eat the food you wanna eat. Still drink the things you want to drink, but here's where the big test comes. You have to pick what empty calories you want. When you're in between your window of eating in the evening, that being said if you like to dabble in your bourbon and beers, you gotta know that is negative calorie intake going into your body. Unfortunately with the bourbons and the nice cold beers there's anywhere from 80 to 400 calories in each serving. Same goes for soda. You have to take that into mind. When you were trying to beat your calorie intake, you don't want to go crazy and eat everything in the world but you could. If you wanted. As long as you shut that window off of not eating late night through the morning. Through the afternoon once you hit that 3 o'clock mark do whatever you enjoy. Eat it all or if you can push yourself and wait till 5,6,7,8 PM. Go for it! Do it. Whatever makes you comfortable. It's the small steps of shocking the body into a new lifestyle. Doing the fasting you're not really changing your diet. I love Taco Bell and guess what? I still go to Taco Bell when I need to go to my Taco Bell. unfortunately I don't go to Taco Bell until 4 o'clock because that's when my window starts. Stay away from sugar drinks. Not saying if you love them stay completely away. Just simply try not to over indulge in sugar fueled drinks even in your food window. Try no sugar sodas. Small changes make big results! Yes yes yes there are cheat days on the weekend. Do what you want. Eat what you want do what you want but you will notice on Monday. You will feel a little I called the Shrek syndrome. When you feel a little bigger than normal. Once you've been living this diet for a while it's good to indulge in what you enjoy, Because without enjoying life what's the point. Enjoy enjoy! Yes there will be hard moments. You will get Hangry and feel like you need to hulk smash something. Grab a handful of nuts. Yes, you can break the fast if you're just starting and it starts to hurt and you really need something. Handful of nuts or protein bar that's it don't go crazy. Have an orange, watermelon apple any fruit you want. Just try to get to the window of eating after 3 o'clock because once your body has had those hours. It kind of starts cleansing the system. It starts to do magic and maybe even heal wounds deep inside your body. Not saying that it does all the time, but you may find just by doing the fasting diet in this little attempts of daily fasting will find you feeling so much better especially after doing the power of 100. Everything just comes into play then you have the problem of having to go shopping and get a whole new wardrobe.

Consult with your doctor before starting a diet and workout regiment.

Chapter 12
Wardrobe

Dress as the person you've always been. Let's be honest most of us are hiding in clothes. We're not wearing the clothes we wanna wear because we don't feel like us. We feel like us trapped. Well let yourself out! Start small and start living, Once you start doing the process. You will feel and see the difference within 100 days. You will notice a completely different person after this process you will mentally spiritually and physically be in a better place than where you were 100 days from the beginning. Don't stop it's good to take breaks just don't ever stop being the best you can be. That's what we were always told that's not a lie. You can do it! Now go for it. Go shopping!

Chapter 13
Sleep and Rest

Enjoy your time. Take time to enjoy it. Do what you love. If you like sitting back watching old episodes of friends or the Office sit back and watch Chandler tell us a funny story. Relax. It's OK you need to start sleeping better. Try too, I know it can be hard. If you can at least get seven hours of sleep at night. Your body will thank you. Your body will naturally start to heal itself. That's what happens when you sleeps. It heals wounds helps with the soreness from working out, sleep helps your pituitary gland grow. You got to rest. Take time and treat yourself. Relax. relax. Put your feet up. Enjoy the moment whatever you enjoy doing do it! You have to to enjoy life because that's what's life all about. Small victories and enjoying it. Smile wake up, say thank you and keep on rolling do something you haven't done before. Experience life it's waiting. The main important thing at the end of a busy day is to rest. Sit back in your favorite chair and do what you like put on your favorite song. It doesn't matter as long as you get to enjoy the moment and rest. Try to sleep more. Your body will Thank you, You will feel more alert and ready for the day's adventure When you rise. Just try to relax.

Chapter 14
Sauna

The sauna is a magical place. Personally I think the sauna has helped me drastically. Physical Spiritual, Mentally Sweat out those toxins. In my sauna time, I enjoy to do some of the workouts. Such as push-ups crunches and leg lifts and squats, Planking In the sauna. It gives a little bit more intensity to the work out. The physical demand should only go between 10 to 20 minutes. You have no problem doing that in the sauna then step up and take it up a level. Even if you're just relaxing in the sauna it helps. The main rule is. You gotta do over 20 minutes. No worries you can take breaks. Take breaks once you feel a certain way. Take a break Drink all the fluids you can. Stay over hydrated. Drink fluids, While you're in there stay hydrated. Even use your favorite sports drink. Try to get the non-sugar sports drinks. Extra sugar is not good for the life change you're experiencing, But if love it enjoy it. Remember empty calories you don't need. Use your sports drinks wisely. Just try to get the non-sugar sports drinks the electrolytes in the sports drinks will help you stay hydrated while in the sauna. Hopefully no cramping occurs, If cramping occurs it happens sometimes step out. Consume as much water as you can to get hydrated. You will drink more water than you've ever thought you could drink before. Please try to drink anywhere from 60 ounces to 120 ounces of water in a day. By doing this it helps your system not feel fatigued. "Hydration is key". Adam Sandler The Water boy. Please step out of the sauna and soak your head in cold water. Shock your body by doing this, you will be able to find different parts of you. That you didn't know exist. You will have conversations with yourself. You can refocus solve situations and problems. Even giving yourself positive affirmations. While you're in there you can get your next dream. You might even meet your new best friend. The sauna has become more of a communal area. A lot of people get together in the sauna after they've worked out or beforehand. The main thing I've noticed is, when you're in the sauna it's almost like a club. there is always someone else you can relate with and talk. It helps even if you want to go in the sauna, play your favorite music and not talk to anybody. Your gonna be to able to relax. Clear your head get that those personal goals you've been trying to achieve. If you don't like it. Don't do it but if you enjoy it, Go for it! Get your time to enjoy and feel better. Sweat out the toxins. Sweat out the bad Let in the good. Just feel better. Be a better you, the power of 100 will always be with you. Just remember you can do it. Go do it!!!

Chapter 15
Classes

Workout classes do them. Try them all. Have fun with them. Push yourself do as
much as you can. Yes, your first couple of times you may not feel like doing a
workout class. Maybe being around others and having the class instructor give
directions. Help tremendously if you are confused or just starting your journey that's
why workout classes are so good. You can do them at any level. Working out classes
are even good to get your spirits lifted. You want a partner in crime? Go do a body
pump class at your local Y or gym. You will meet all kinds of great people in classes.
Do it . Have fun try a spin class try anything just push yourself to do new things.
Remember that goes for life too. Whatever you enjoy do it. Do what makes you
happy, because what we've learned by getting older is. No one else is going to make
us happy. We need to make ourselves happy. By making ourselves happy maybe we
can pass on that happiness to others as they see, we're living happy bringing peace of
mind. Have fun accept a new challenge. Search and find what works for you. There is
no law in this lifestyle change. By doing a new class taking your body and spirit to a
new level. You're doing something you've never done before. Congratulations!
Please try something new have fun with it. Sweat it out. Leave it in there. I personally
take the mindset of Richard Simmons, having fun enjoying everything as I can. Don't
be shy get up and dance be a goofball it helps. You're building a better you for you.
Have fun smile more. Most important enjoy the journey. Try a class.

Chapter 16
100 Days

100 days have passed. After this hundred days you should be a new person. You should be on a path to continuing to grow. Continuing to get better. Continuing with your goals. You might not have reached your goal in the hundred days. Guess what you're halfway there. That's all that matters. Don't stop. Keep on believing in yourself , you're the best person for you. You can do anything. You just gotta go for it. I believe in you and you believe in you. Say it out loud say it proud. I'm ready let's go! I'M READY LET'S GO! I'M READY LET'S GO!

Get excited. Stay excited every day in your journey. Every day is a new moment. Enjoy it! Embrace it. Say thank you to everyone. Say hello to everyone make someone else's day. Be an inspiration that people didn't know they needed. You're the best!Thank you for taking the time to improve yourself. Keep on going for it never stop. You're the best!

"Dream. Dream BIG! Make your life your dream."
S.M.

<u>Goals Dreams and Progression</u>
<u>Write your Goals and Dreams.</u>
<u>Make it happen. 100 times…</u>

www.ingramcontent.com/pod-product-compliance
Lightning Source LLC
Chambersburg PA
CBHW081605250726
48653CB00009B/3567